Weight Loss Compass

The truth about Fat, Fitness and Lasting Change

Table of Contents

Chapter 1: Foreword.. 1

Chapter 2: Introduction 5

Chapter 3: Life Before Abundance: How Humans Thrived Before Agriculture and Industry.................. 9

Chapter 4: The Evolutionary Machine — How the Human Body is Built for Survival............................ 19

Chapter 5: Secrets of Longevity: Ancient Wisdom and Modern Insights from Long-Living Cultures 35

Chapter 6: The Rhythm of Nourishment: Feeding, Fasting, and the Metabolic Journey 39

Chapter 7: Mathematics of Fasting.......................... 67

Chapter 8: A-Ha moment and Hard Truths 71

Chapter 9: What does it all mean? Let's talk about the 'How' of weight loss and healthy living... 75

Chapter 10: The Final Weigh-In: What It All Comes Down To...81

References 85

Chapter 1: Foreword

At my annual wellness check, my doctor mentioned my slightly elevated A1C and cholesterol. While my EKG was fine, my weight still flagged as overweight, despite last year's 25-pound loss. Progress is progress, I thought—but then my doctor made a surprising suggestion.

Then my doctor hit me with it: *"I can prescribe Ozempic for you. It'll help you lose the excess weight."*

I paused.

"'Are these drugs safe?' I asked my doctor, curious but wary. His response intrigued me: *'They mimic hormones that signal fullness, slowing digestion—essentially mimicking bariatric surgery without the scalpel.'*

This simple explanation sparked my curiosity: could I mimic these effects naturally?

Okay, I thought. So basically, it tricks you into eating less and less often.

"Why can't I just do that myself, without the risks?" I asked.

My doctor smiled.

"You could," he admitted. *"But most people don't have the mental strength to stick with it long term."*

And that right there was the seed for this book. I declined the Ozempic prescription and instead asked myself a far more interesting question:

"Why hasn't any diet I've tried actually worked?"

I've struggled with my weight for as long as I can remember. Losing my thyroid—thanks to its impressive size and a flair for cancer risk—didn't do me any favors. Over the past decade, I've tried every diet under the sun. Some worked for a while; others were complete flops. But no matter how promising they seemed, the weight always crept back.

After that doctor's visit, I started obsessing over two questions: *Why do we get obese in the first place?* and *Why is our body so determined to hoard fat like it's preparing for the apocalypse?* Frustrated—and fueled by curiosity—I went on a research binge, devouring books, podcasts, and scientific articles like my life depended on it.

Luckily, I had a secret weapon: my wife, the brains of the operation. She's got a Ph.D. in pharmaceutical sciences and a history as a research scientist, which made her the perfect person to bounce ideas off. She's also humble enough not to rub it in when she's right (which is most of the time). She reviewed the science in this book with a sharp eye, steering me away from some of my more... let's call them "creative" theories.

With her help and my own knack for tackling new challenges—honed by years of self-teaching skills like golf, darts, and even painting—I started piecing together a clear picture of obesity. Over time, I unearthed a simple, durable set of truths. I didn't stop reading until I was confident I'd looked at the issue from every angle—historical, medical, genetic, and even ancient perspectives.

Writing this book became my way of organizing those truths into a roadmap, one grounded in science but easy enough to follow. My wife deserves a massive shoutout here; her contributions kept this book rooted in reality. Together, we've created something I hope will resonate with you—a guide to weight loss that skips the gimmicks and gets straight to what works.

So, here it is: my "a-ha" moment, captured on paper. I hope it helps you the way it's helped me. Let's do this!

Chapter 2: Introduction

The Weight of the Matter: Why We Need a New Perspective

Weight loss is everywhere—bookstores, social media, morning shows—all promising a magic fix. Yet despite endless solutions, obesity rates keep climbing. Clearly, the standard advice isn't working.

The real problem isn't the weight itself—it's the mismatch between our ancient biology and today's environment. For millennia, we adapted to scarcity, relying on physical labor and unpredictable food supplies to survive.

If we want real progress, we need a fresh perspective— one that's rooted in science and embraces the quirks and complexities of our bodies. It's about truly understanding how our bodies work, why they cling to fat like a toddler with a favorite blanket, and how we can align our health goals with our physiology instead of constantly waging war against it.

This is not your traditional weight-loss advice. We're diving into the science—evolutionary, genetic, and lifestyle factors—to uncover what really works. This isn't just another guide to shed a few pounds. It's for those ready to break free from the endless cycle of diets, failures, and frustrations. Because when it comes to weight loss, knowledge isn't just power—it's your ticket out of the hamster wheel of hopelessness and into a sustainable, healthier life. Let's get to it.

Unpacking the Science of Weight

When it comes to weight loss, the advice often boils down to the world's least helpful soundbite: *"Eat less."* If someone's feeling extra insightful, they might tack on *"Move more."* Simple, right? Except, if it were that simple, we wouldn't have an entire industry built around weight-loss books, fad diets, fitness gadgets, and miracle supplements. Clearly, something more complicated is going on. Spoiler: weight regulation isn't just about willpower or counting calories. It's about biology, genetics, psychology, and the evolutionary quirks that got us here.

Let's pop the hood and take a closer look. Our bodies aren't designed for your Instagram fitness goals; they're designed for survival. For most of human history, food was scarce, and our bodies got really good at storing fat to ride out the tough times. Fast forward to the modern buffet of caloric abundance, and guess what? Our bodies are still hoarding fat like a squirrel stashing nuts for a winter that never comes.

But that's just the beginning. Each of us has our own genetic blueprint that affects how we store and use energy. Some people burn calories like a bonfire; others hold onto them as if prepping for an ice age. Hormones, too, play a starring role—dictating hunger, fullness, and even how you feel about that chocolate cake calling your name. And then there's your gut microbiome, the unsung hero (or villain) of weight regulation. Those trillions of microscopic critters in your digestive tract don't just digest food—they influence your cravings, metabolism, and how your body processes fat. It's like having an invisible committee voting on your every snack choice.

We're leaving behind the myths that blame weight gain on a lack of willpower or a single "bad" food choice. Instead, we're diving into the science that reveals the unique factors shaping each person's experience with weight.

The Blueprint for Change: What This Book Will—and Won't—Promise

What this book *does* promise is a fresh perspective on weight—one rooted in science, sustainability, and a genuine respect for the body's natural design. Think of it as a roadmap, one that digs into the "why" behind the "what." Why does the body cling to fat like it's planning for an apocalypse? Why do so many weight-loss methods fall flat, and why do some approaches work better for certain people? Armed with these insights, you'll be equipped to make informed, gimmick-free decisions based on understanding, not desperation.

Once we've unpacked the "why" behind weight gain and obesity, we'll move on to the "how" of addressing it. You'll learn how to build your own plan, tailored to your unique biology, habits, and goals. I'll guide you through the levers you can control to create lasting change—no one-size-fits-all solutions here.

The best solutions are often the ones that respect your body's innate wisdom. No fads. No empty promises. Just an informed, practical path forward.

Oh, and one more thing—the statutory warning. While the science in this book is rigorously vetted and as comprehensive as possible, I'm not a medical professional. This is your health we're talking about, so when you create your own plan based on what you learn here, make sure to consult your doctor. They'll help you align your plan with any medications, health conditions, or other individual factors.

Now, let's dive in!

Chapter 3: Life Before Abundance: How Humans Thrived Before Agriculture and Industry

Hunter-Gatherer Days: Survival and Adaptation

Life as a hunter-gatherer had no alarms or notifications—but also no stocked pantry. Breakfast wasn't waiting; it was running on four legs or hanging from a tree. Eating required effort, and every meal was earned. This was the daily grind for our ancestors, and it shaped us in ways that still echo in our lives today.

For early humans, survival was an all-day, every-day affair. Hunting and gathering weren't weekend hobbies; they were the only way to stay alive. Long treks across rugged landscapes, tracking game, and foraging for berries, nuts, and roots made up their daily itinerary. Forget three square meals or snack breaks—they ate when they could and what they could, turning meals into opportunistic jackpots rather than scheduled events. If that sounds exhausting, that's because it was. Movement wasn't optional, and the modern concept of "exercise" didn't exist because, frankly, it didn't need to. Staying active was simply part of the deal.

But here's the fascinating part: this feast-or-famine lifestyle left a mark that we still carry today. Our ancestors didn't have a guaranteed food supply. Some days, they hit the culinary jackpot with a successful hunt; other days, they scraped by on whatever they could forage. To navigate unpredictable food supplies, our ancestors evolved to store energy as fat—a lifesaving insurance policy during lean times.

This cycle of "search, feast, survive" wired our metabolic systems to prioritize storing calories over burning them. In a world where the next meal was never certain, every ounce of fat mattered. Our bodies became incredibly efficient at conserving energy, treating fat as a prized resource, not a problem. Fast forward to today: we've swapped hunting grounds for grocery aisles and foraging for food delivery apps, but our bodies haven't gotten the memo. They're still running the same ancient program, prioritizing storage like we're one missed meal away from disaster.

Understanding this ancestral setup helps us make sense of the weight challenges we face in the modern world. Our biology is still playing by the rules of a game that ended thousands of years ago, stuck in survival mode while we swim in a sea of caloric abundance. This isn't just a quirky historical tidbit; it's a crucial piece of the puzzle. Our bodies are responding exactly as they're designed to—still ready for the hunt, even if the only thing we're chasing is the pizza delivery guy.

Feast and Famine: The Natural Cycle of Scarcity

In the world of early humans, life didn't come with the convenience of a pantry or fridge. Food wasn't waiting in the cupboard or freezer; it was out there—wild, unpredictable, and often maddeningly elusive. This meant our ancestors lived through cycles of plenty followed by periods of scarcity. They didn't count calories or stress about balanced diets; they ate whatever they could, whenever they could, adapting to whatever nature provided. This feast-or-famine rhythm wasn't just a survival strategy—it became a defining force in shaping human physiology.

When the going was good—after a successful hunt or a seasonal harvest—early humans feasted, packing in calories like there was no tomorrow (because, quite literally, there might not be). The body, ever the diligent prepper, shifted into storage mode, turning those extra calories into fat reserves. During lean times, these fat stores became their lifeline, providing the energy they needed to make it through the next drought, winter, or string of failed hunts. This wasn't just a clever adaptation; it was a survival superpower.

Fast forward to today, and the idea of feast-or-famine sounds more like a bad dream than a way of life. We're surrounded by a near-endless supply of food, available at the tap of a screen or the turn of a corner. But here's the kicker: our bodies haven't moved on. They're still running on the same ancient software, reacting to every calorie as if a famine is lurking just around the bend. Every bite we take kicks off those same fat-storing mechanisms that once protected our ancestors from starvation. The problem? That famine never comes.

This evolutionary hangover helps explain why losing weight can feel like fighting an uphill battle. Our bodies are designed to conserve energy, not to give it up easily. When we cut calories or skip meals, the body doesn't throw a party; it slows down metabolism and hoards fat, assuming we're entering another famine. This is why crash diets often backfire, leaving us frustrated while our bodies cling to fat like it's the last can of beans on the shelf.

Here's the irony: the very mechanism that kept our ancestors alive is now working against us. In a world of constant food availability, we're battling biology that's stuck in survival mode. But instead of trying to outsmart our bodies with extreme diets, what if we worked with them instead?

Physical Activity as a Necessity: Movement in the Ancient World

For our hunter-gatherer ancestors, physical activity wasn't a choice—it was survival. There were no gym memberships, yoga mats, or step-counting apps. Every movement served a purpose: gathering food, hunting prey, building shelters, hauling supplies, or trekking to the next campsite. Exercise, as we know it, didn't exist.

Movement was life, as essential and automatic as breathing.

They didn't spend their days parked behind desks or slouched on couches bingeing the Paleolithic version of Netflix (spoiler: it didn't exist). Sedentary wasn't an option because survival demanded mobility. Studies suggest these early humans clocked in several miles of walking daily—not because they had fitness goals, but because that's what it took to find food and stay alive. Sprinting after animals, climbing trees for fruit, and hauling firewood were just part of the routine. Their muscles were strong, their endurance impressive, and their agility remarkable—all built naturally by necessity, not choice.

This nonstop movement didn't just keep them alive; it profoundly shaped their health. Physical activity supported their cardiovascular fitness, strengthened muscles, and kept their metabolism humming along at a steady clip. Calories were burned not just in bursts of activity but even at rest. Movement also acted as a natural appetite regulator, syncing energy intake with energy expenditure. Food wasn't just fuel—it was earned, and the balance between eating and moving was baked into their way of life.

Fast forward to today, and we've traded mobility for modern conveniences. Tasks that once required effort have been outsourced to machines, apps, and gadgets, leaving us with a lifestyle our ancestors would barely recognize. Now, we have to pencil in "exercise" as a separate activity, a chore squeezed into busy schedules. Ironically, this structured exercise often feels like a fight against our evolutionary tendency to conserve energy when it's not needed.

While our modern lives have become sedentary, our bodies haven't caught up. They're still hardwired for movement. Without regular activity, our metabolism slows, muscle mass diminishes, and our bodies begin storing fat like they're prepping for a rainy season. Insulin resistance creeps in, and energy balance goes haywire.

The good news? We can reclaim this ancient wisdom by rethinking how we view movement. It's not just about hitting calorie targets or crushing fitness goals; it's about fulfilling a basic biological need. Moving regularly isn't a luxury—it's essential for keeping our bodies functioning as they were designed to. And it doesn't have to mean grueling gym sessions. By weaving consistent activity into our daily lives—taking the stairs, walking more, or simply staying on our feet longer—we're honoring our evolutionary blueprint. In doing so, we move closer to achieving the balance our bodies have been craving all along.

Nutritional Realities: What Our Ancestors Really Ate

Our hunter-gatherer ancestors weren't chowing down on burgers, spaghetti, or protein bars. Their diets weren't crafted with "macros" in mind or guided by trendy nutrition plans. Instead, they ate whatever they could find, hunt, or catch—because survival didn't come with a menu. Food availability depended on the season, location, and a fair amount of luck. The concept of "low-carb" or "high-protein" meals? Not on their radar. Their priority was simple: find food and make it to the next day.

The hunter-gatherer diet was as varied as the landscapes they roamed. It was naturally nutrient-dense and comprised plants, animals, nuts, seeds, roots, and fruits. Carbohydrates came from fibrous roots, berries, and wild fruits—not the refined sugars and processed grains we know today. These carbs were packed with fiber, leading to slower digestion, steady energy levels, and better blood sugar regulation. Protein came from wild game, fish, and even insects, while fats were sourced from animals, nuts, and seeds. Unlike the calorie-dense processed foods of modern times, their meals were low in calories but rich in essential nutrients, providing the vitamins and minerals they needed to thrive.

Calories were harder to come by back then. This wasn't a world of abundance—it was a world of necessity. Food was often scarce, and their bodies adapted by becoming exceptionally efficient at extracting and storing energy. When they hit the jackpot with a successful hunt or a rare trove of calorie-rich food, it was feast time. But regular, large meals were not part of the deal.

Fiber-rich plants made up a big portion of their diet, bringing benefits we're just beginning to fully appreciate.

These fibrous foods kept them full, supported gut health, and naturally limited how much energy their bodies stored as fat. Plants also provided a treasure trove of antioxidants and micronutrients, bolstering their immune systems and overall health. Animal foods, when available, delivered the protein and fats crucial for brain development, muscle repair, and energy reserves. The balance of carbs, fats, and protein wasn't a calculated choice—it was dictated by nature.

What does this mean for us in the age of food delivery apps and 24/7 grocery stores? While we don't need to forage in the forest or eat like we're prepping for a famine, understanding what our bodies evolved to thrive on can guide us toward smarter choices. Our ancestors ate in sync with their biology, and their diets supported balanced energy, hormone regulation, and efficient metabolism. Our ancestors' bodies evolved over millions of years to adapt to the food available to them. Their diet wasn't a matter of choice—it was dictated by necessity. In contrast, we live in a world of abundance, which means we must make conscious decisions about what we eat and when we eat it. By opting for nutrient-dense, whole foods in our own diets, we can tap into the same principles and give our bodies what they're naturally designed for.

Our bodies haven't forgotten their ancient roots. They still function best on real, unprocessed foods that nourish rather than overwhelm. Looking back at our ancestors' diets offers valuable insight—not as a template to copy exactly, but as a reminder to respect our biology.

The Evolutionary Advantage of Fat: Why Our Bodies Were Built to Store

Fat often gets a bad rap in today's weight-obsessed culture, but for our ancestors, it was a lifesaver—a built-in survival tool that kept them alive through the leanest times. In the grand story of human evolution, fat wasn't a design flaw; it was a stroke of genius. Think of it as the ultimate CD (Certificate of Deposit): calories deposited during times of plenty and withdrawn when food was scarce. Without this ingenious system, early humans wouldn't have stood a chance during the countless famines and food shortages that shaped their existence.

Picture going days without a successful hunt or foraging haul. Without fat reserves, energy would have run out quickly, leaving early humans vulnerable to starvation. But thanks to the body's ability to store fat, they could pack away surplus calories during good times and draw on that energy later, powering them through the tough days. This adaptability wasn't just a nifty trick—it was a game-changing adaptation that made humans resilient and capable of thriving in harsh, unpredictable environments.

Even today, our bodies are remarkably good at this. When we consume more energy than we immediately need, our body doesn't toss it out—it saves it for later. Through a process called **lipogenesis**, extra calories, particularly from carbs and fats, are converted into triglycerides and tucked away in fat cells. These cells are like overachievers at work; they can expand and multiply, giving our bodies a near-limitless ability to store energy. When food gets scarce, **lipolysis** kicks in, breaking down those fat reserves into usable fuel to keep us alive and moving.

What was once an evolutionary advantage has turned into a modern challenge. Fat storage, designed to save our ancestors, now works against us in a world where food is cheap, sedentary lifestyles are the norm, and movement is optional. Our bodies still see fat as a valuable resource, not an aesthetic problem or a fitness hurdle. They're focused on survival, not your goal weight.

Recognizing fat storage as an evolutionary solution—not a personal failing—can completely change how we approach weight and health. It's not about battling your body or blaming yourself; it's about understanding that your body is doing exactly what it was designed to do. By aligning our diet and lifestyle with this biological reality, we can work *with* our bodies instead of fighting against them. Fat isn't the villain in this story—it's an ancient solution to an ancient problem. The real challenge now is finding a way to honor that legacy in a world where scarcity has been replaced by surplus.

Chapter 4: The Evolutionary Machine — How the Human Body is Built for Survival

Sun-Up to Sundown: A Typical Day in the Life of the 5000 B.C.E. Human

Sunrise - The Natural Alarm Clock

Before the days of alarms blaring and coffee brewing, nature had the job of waking us up. For early humans, dawn's first light was the cue to rise, naturally syncing their internal clocks with the day-night cycle. Their morning rituals were practical—fetching water, stoking the fire, or tending to livestock if they had any. No doom-scrolling through social media; instead, exposure to sunlight jump-started their day, regulating their circadian rhythms and providing a natural energy boost.

Breakfast wasn't a lavish feast; it was a quick, practical affair. A handful of nuts, some fresh berries, or a piece of dried meat left over from the previous day was enough to fuel the morning's activities. These foods were portable, nutrient-dense, and required no prep—perfect for a lifestyle that revolved around efficiency and survival. This light morning meal kept them energized for early tasks without slowing them down, embodying the ultimate "grab-and-go" breakfast long before smoothies and protein bars hit the scene.

Mid-Morning Fitness

The real exercise of the day kicked in by mid-morning, as survival demanded physical effort. Gathering firewood, foraging, or—if they were part of an agricultural society—tending crops and livestock required functional, full-body movement. For hunters, this could also mean tracking prey, complete with bursts of sprinting. These weren't leisurely tasks; they ranged from moderate to intense, involving walking, lifting, bending, climbing, and occasionally running. No gym memberships or targeted bicep curls here—every muscle group got a workout, and endurance naturally developed through these varied daily activities. In short, their lives were one continuous outdoor boot camp, designed by necessity.

Noon: The Big Midday Meal

By midday, it was time for the largest meal of the day. A typical spread might feature grains, vegetables, roots, and, if it had been a lucky day, some fish or small game. Meals were hearty but simple, often dominated by plant-based ingredients that were in season. Processed snacks? Not an option. Their diet was naturally high in fiber and low in sugar, supporting gut health and maintaining steady energy levels. This midday meal was as much about fueling the body as it was about replenishing energy for the tasks still ahead.

Early Afternoon: Rest and Recharge

As the midday sun peaked, early humans often paused for a short rest or social break, especially in warmer climates. This was the time to relax, chat, or take care of lighter tasks like weaving or repairing tools. It wasn't just a luxury; this downtime served a practical purpose, letting them recharge while avoiding the heat of the day. Think of it as an ancient version of the siesta—a natural rhythm that kept them refreshed and ready to tackle whatever the rest of the afternoon demanded.

Afternoon - Functional Movement Continues

The afternoon tasks like crafting tools, gathering food, or prepping for the evening meal. Physical activity levels were lower than in the morning but still constant, providing a balanced, varied workout throughout the day. The goal was functional fitness, not aesthetics, and every movement had a purpose tied to survival.

Sunset - Family and Community Time

As evening approached, everyone prepared for a meal that was typically lighter—maybe leftovers from earlier or a simple dish with whatever was available. This meal was about togetherness, with family or the community gathering to share stories, trade knowledge, and bond. Without artificial light, the day's pace naturally slowed, creating a wind-down routine that prepared them for restful sleep.

Night - Segmented Sleep, the Pre-Modern Way

Sleep came early, often right after sunset. Pre-modern humans followed a pattern known as **segmented sleep**, where they slept in two distinct phases with a quiet period of wakefulness in between. This break in the night was used for meditation, quiet activities, or even a snack, before going back to bed until dawn. The natural darkness and absence of artificial light supported deep, restorative sleep, allowing them to wake up refreshed and ready for another active day.

Summary

In a day, our pre-modern human walked thousands of steps across varied terrain, lifted natural weights and lived in alignment with the earth's rhythms. Their diet was simple and whole, with meals timed according to availability rather than schedules. Every aspect of their day, from sun-up to sundown, was designed to keep them naturally fit, connected, and aligned with their environment.

On many occasions they also faced periods of food scarcity where they had to survive on little or no food for days (if not weeks).

Over millions of years, through survival-for-the fittest, our body was built to live in this world.

Modern day humans are fundamentally the same as these pre-modern humans. So, Let's understand this machine better.

The Metabolic Engine: How Our Bodies Process and Store Energy

Our bodies are, at their core, marvelously efficient machines, evolved through millennia to make the most out of every bite. The human metabolic engine is finely tuned to convert food into energy, store any surplus for later use, and keep everything running smoothly. And when it comes to survival, the body's motto could be summed up as, "Waste not, want not."

The journey of food through our bodies is a sophisticated process. When we eat, our digestive system breaks down carbohydrates, fats, and proteins into their simplest forms—glucose, fatty acids, and amino acids. These components are then absorbed into the bloodstream, becoming fuel for immediate energy needs. Glucose is the body's favorite quick-energy source, rapidly supplying our cells, muscles, and brain with the fuel they need to operate.

But what happens when we eat more than we need? Here's where the body's "savings account" kicks in. Any glucose that isn't immediately used gets stored as glycogen in the liver and muscles. This glycogen acts as a short-term energy reserve, ready to be called on when we need a quick boost. Once the glycogen stores are full, however, the body has another trick up its sleeve: it converts the excess glucose into fat (like a CD), storing it in adipose tissue for long-term use.

The process doesn't stop there. Fats from our diet have their own journey. After digestion, fatty acids are shuttled into fat cells, where they're stored as triglycerides. Unlike glycogen, which is limited in storage capacity, fat cells can expand and even multiply, providing the body with almost limitless storage. This is an evolutionary advantage; in a world where the next meal was never guaranteed, being able to store energy as fat meant having reserves to survive periods of scarcity.

Every extra calorie, every unburned gram of glucose, has the potential to become stored energy—energy our bodies assume we might need later.

Hormones and Hunger: The Signals That Drive Eating and Energy Use

If you've ever felt like your appetite has a mind of its own, you're not far off. The body is constantly fine-tuning hunger and fullness signals, orchestrated by a complex network of hormones that keep us from starving—or from overeating, at least in theory. Hormones like insulin, ghrelin, and leptin are the unsung heroes (or sometimes villains) in this story, working behind the scenes to regulate energy balance and ensure that we have enough fuel to survive.

Let's start with insulin, the "storage hormone." After we eat, insulin is released by the pancreas to help shuttle glucose from our bloodstream into cells where it can be used for energy. Any leftover glucose is converted to glycogen or, when those stores are full, to fat. Insulin doesn't just manage glucose; it also signals the body to store energy, making it essential in the body's fat-storage strategy. When insulin levels are high, the body shifts into storage mode. But chronically high insulin levels, common in diets heavy in processed carbs and sugars, can lead to insulin resistance—a state in which the body struggles to regulate blood sugar, often contributing to weight gain and obesity.

Then there's ghrelin, known as the "hunger hormone." Ghrelin levels spike when the stomach is empty, sending signals to the brain that it's time to eat. In a sense, ghrelin is your body's alarm system, making sure you seek out food when energy stores are low. It's a hormone finely attuned to survival, a natural prompt to fill up and store energy. Unfortunately, in a world where food is constantly available, ghrelin doesn't always know when to quit. Even after a large meal, ghrelin levels can rise again when the body senses the slightest deficit, urging you to keep eating just in case.

On the flip side, we have leptin, the "satiety hormone." Produced by fat cells, leptin's job is to tell the brain when energy stores are sufficient, signaling fullness and reducing appetite. The more fat cells you have, the more leptin is released, which in theory should curb hunger. But here's the kicker: in people with higher levels of body fat, leptin often doesn't work as it should. The brain can become resistant to leptin's message, leaving hunger signals unchecked despite ample fat stores. It's a bit like having a full tank of gas but your car's fuel gauge still flashes empty.

Together, these hormones form a feedback loop that regulates when we feel hungry or full. In an ideal world, ghrelin would make us hungry when we need energy, insulin would help us store any excess, and leptin would signal when we're full. But modern diets, stress, and lifestyle habits can throw this system off balance, leading to chronic hunger, frequent cravings, and relentless fat storage.

This hormonal tug-of-war highlights why weight management is rarely as simple as "eat less, move more." When these signals are misaligned, the body resists calorie deficits, interpreting them as threats to survival. Hormones like ghrelin and leptin are programmed for survival, not waistlines, meaning our efforts to restrict calories can sometimes lead to greater hunger, slowed metabolism, and even more fat storage.

The Role of Fat: Why the Body Treats Fat as a Precious Resource

The science of fat is surprisingly elegant. When we eat more calories than we immediately need, the body doesn't waste the excess; it stores it as fat for later use. This stored fat can then be broken down into fatty acids and glycerol through a process called lipolysis when energy is needed but food isn't available. Fat storage, from a biological perspective, is a high-yield savings account that the body can tap into during "financial crises" like fasting, extended exercise, or periods of food scarcity. It's not just efficient; it's essential for long-term survival.

What's remarkable is how efficient fat is as an energy source. Each gram of fat provides roughly 9 calories, more than double what carbohydrates and proteins offer. This high energy density means that the body can store a significant amount of energy in a relatively small amount of space. Fat cells, known as adipocytes, are incredibly adaptable. They can expand to store more fat and even multiply when needed, ensuring that the body has ample storage capacity for times when food might be in short supply.

But fat does more than just store energy; it also plays several crucial roles in keeping our bodies functioning smoothly. Fat helps insulate our bodies, regulate temperature, protect vital organs, and even support hormone production. Some hormones, like leptin, are actually produced by fat cells, which means fat directly influences our energy balance and appetite. Fat is also essential for absorbing fat-soluble vitamins (A, D, E, and K), supporting cell structure, and maintaining a healthy nervous system. It's no exaggeration to say that fat is one of the body's most versatile and vital assets.

So, if fat is so essential, why does it get such a bad reputation today? The problem isn't fat itself; it's the excess of it, made possible by our modern environment of abundant, calorie-dense foods and minimal physical exertion. In a world where food is plentiful and we spend much of our day sitting, fat storage has gone from an asset to a liability. Our bodies are still operating on the ancient assumption that food might be scarce, diligently storing away extra calories in case of a future famine. But that famine never comes.

The Thrifty Gene Hypothesis: Built to Survive, Not to Stay Lean

Why does it feel like some people can eat anything they want and stay thin while others seem to gain weight just looking at dessert? The answer may lie in what's known as the "thrifty gene hypothesis." This theory suggests that certain genes in our DNA make some of us naturally better at storing fat. Far from being a curse, these genes were once critical to human survival—they were the ultimate insurance policy for getting through tough times.

In the environment our ancestors faced, food was anything but predictable. Over generations, people with genes that allowed them to store fat efficiently had an advantage: they could build up energy reserves during times of abundance and tap into those reserves when food was scarce. In other words, they were genetically programmed to be "thrifty" with their calories, holding onto every bit of energy to increase their chances of survival.

The thrifty gene hypothesis suggests that this tendency to store fat is built into our genetic code. For most of human history, these genes were essential, enabling people to endure long winters, droughts, or periods of migration without constantly needing to find food.

What's particularly challenging is that the thrifty gene effect isn't uniform. Not everyone has the same level of "thriftiness." Some people are more genetically inclined to store fat, while others naturally burn through calories faster. This is why different people respond to the same diet or exercise regimen in different ways. For those with thrifty genes, it's simply harder to lose weight and keep it off, as their bodies are actively working to conserve energy, even in a food-rich environment.

This genetic tendency to store fat is not just about survival, though; it also impacts the way we respond to hunger and fullness. Thrifty genes are often accompanied by heightened hunger signals and a slower metabolism. These traits, once essential for survival, make weight loss and maintenance challenging in today's world. When we try to lose weight, these genes send out signals that we're entering a famine, prompting the body to reduce energy expenditure and increase hunger—both strategies to encourage fat storage. The result is a biological tug-of-war that can make dieting feel like an uphill battle.

The Brain-Body Connection: How the Mind and Metabolism Work Together

If you've ever felt like your body has a mind of its own, you're not entirely wrong. The brain plays an enormous role in regulating our metabolism, hunger, and overall energy balance. It's the command center, monitoring what's going on in the body and sending out signals to ensure that we're well-fueled, well-protected, and, in its eyes, well-prepared to survive. From hunger pangs to cravings to the feeling of fullness after a meal, much of what we experience as "instinct" or "willpower" actually originates in the brain.

The brain, specifically the hypothalamus, is responsible for managing energy balance. It's constantly processing information from the body about energy stores, nutrient intake, and metabolic demands. When the brain senses that energy levels are low—say, when we're in a calorie deficit or skipping meals—it responds by increasing hunger hormones like ghrelin to encourage eating. Conversely, when energy levels are high, it releases satiety hormones to curb appetite. This intricate feedback system helps maintain homeostasis, or balance, in the body. But here's the catch: it's all based on survival, not weight loss.

One of the brain's primary responsibilities is to protect us from starvation. If food intake is restricted, the brain doesn't see it as a voluntary diet; it interprets it as a potential famine. In response, it activates a series of mechanisms to conserve energy, including slowing metabolism and increasing hunger. This is why, after a period of dieting, it's common to feel hungrier and have a harder time resisting food. The brain is simply trying to bring energy reserves back to a level it considers safe.

The brain also plays a significant role in cravings and reward-driven eating. The release of dopamine—a feel-good neurotransmitter—is triggered by food, especially high-calorie foods rich in sugar and fat. This isn't a design flaw; it's another survival strategy. In times when food was scarce, rewarding high-calorie foods helped early humans seek out nutrient-dense sources of energy. Today, though, with high-calorie foods everywhere, this reward system can backfire, leading to cravings that feel impossible to resist.

Stress is another area where the brain-body connection shows its power. When we're stressed, the brain releases cortisol, a hormone that prompts the body to store more fat, particularly around the abdomen. This, too, is a survival strategy. In ancient times, stress often meant physical danger or a shortage of resources, so storing fat in response to stress was a way to prepare for tough times. Unfortunately, modern stressors like work deadlines or financial worries activate the same response, pushing the body to store fat even when physical danger is nowhere in sight.

The brain's involvement doesn't end with survival instincts; it also impacts the way we perceive food, hunger, and satisfaction. Studies have shown that visual cues, emotional associations, and even the memory of a recent meal can influence hunger and eating behaviors. The brain's interpretation of these signals often overrides actual physical hunger, making us more likely to eat based on habit, mood, or social setting rather than true need.

We're not just dealing with biology; we're dealing with deeply ingrained survival instincts and reward systems that are built to keep us alive, not to keep us slim. By learning to recognize these signals and understanding the reasons behind them, we can start working with our brain rather than fighting against it.

Adaptation Over Aesthetics: Why Our Bodies Aren't Programmed for Six-Packs

If our bodies had a mission statement, it would go something like this: ***Survival first, aesthetics later... or maybe never***. For better or worse, our biology has a pretty straightforward goal: keep us alive and thriving in a world full of unpredictable challenges. The six-pack abs and lean physique idealized in modern culture were never part of the survival package. Instead, our bodies evolved with a laser focus on efficiency, adaptability, and the ability to store energy—not on fitting into skinny jeans.

The human body prioritizes functions that ensure survival: immune support, tissue repair, reproductive health, and energy conservation. When energy is limited, the body prioritizes these essential functions, putting muscle tone and lean body composition on the back burner. Having a low percentage of body fat, while it might look impressive on magazine covers, actually signals to the body that resources might be limited, triggering mechanisms to conserve fat stores and reduce energy output. This is why achieving and maintaining a very low body fat percentage can feel like a constant battle; it's simply not what the body was designed to do.

Additionally, lean muscle mass and visible muscle definition are not as essential for survival as one might think. Muscles require a lot of energy to maintain, and in an environment of scarcity, carrying extra muscle without the fat to fuel it would have been a liability. Muscles built for strength and endurance were more useful than those meant for aesthetics. Our ancestors' bodies were optimized for function, not form. The body's goal was to be fit enough to hunt, gather, and survive, not to be photo-ready.

Modern fitness goals, with their focus on muscle definition and fat reduction, often require overriding natural bodily instincts. Achieving a "cut" physique goes against the body's natural inclination to store fat as a backup fuel source. In fact, when body fat drops to very low levels, the body often triggers responses like increased hunger, decreased metabolism, and even hormonal changes to encourage fat storage. These mechanisms evolved to protect us, but they can make maintaining a low body fat percentage feel like fighting against our biology.

It's important to understand that the ideals of lean muscle and low body fat are cultural constructs, not biological imperatives. The human body is adaptable, yes, but it's designed for practical survival rather than modern-day fitness standards. This perspective can help us adopt a more balanced approach to health and fitness, one that respects our biology rather than constantly challenging it.

Chapter 5: Secrets of Longevity: Ancient Wisdom and Modern Insights from Long-Living Cultures

Throughout history, people have marveled at certain regions where reaching a ripe old age seems to be the norm. Known as "Blue Zones," these areas have drawn researchers, journalists, and health enthusiasts alike to uncover the secrets behind their residents' remarkable longevity. Let's dive into the lifestyle habits, food routines, and fasting practices of these long-living cultures, with insights from Ayurveda adding depth to our understanding of health and well-being.

Blue Zones: Where Living Long is the norm

Research has identified several "Blue Zones" around the world where centenarians (people living beyond 100 years) are unusually common. These include Okinawa in Japan, Sardinia in Italy, Nicoya Peninsula in Costa Rica, Ikaria in Greece, and a Seventh-Day Adventist community in Loma Linda, California. So, what do these regions have in common?

Residents of Blue Zones tend to eat primarily plant-based diets rich in vegetables, legumes, and whole grains. They also consume moderate amounts of dairy, like goat's milk in Sardinia, and fish, like in Okinawa, but keep red meat and processed foods to a minimum. Their diet isn't the only thing they share; other factors like daily physical activity (typically embedded in daily tasks), strong social connections, and a sense of purpose are key contributors to their longevity.

Fasting practices are also a common thread. For instance, many residents of Ikaria practice intermittent fasting as part of their Greek Orthodox faith, with fasting days sprinkled throughout the calendar year. This fasting aligns well with the natural rhythm of their diet and daily life, providing a chance for the body to rest and rejuvenate.

The Power of Fasting: Ancient Rituals for Health and Longevity

Fasting isn't new, and it isn't just trendy. Nearly every culture has a tradition of fasting that's tied to spiritual practices and, surprisingly, aligns with modern insights into metabolic health. Here's a look at some notable fasting practices around the world:

- **Jain Ayambil Fasting:** In this structured fast, Jains avoid foods with spices, oils, and sugars, eating only simple, unprocessed meals. This practice is said to aid in detoxification, reduce inflammation, and improve mental clarity
- **Orthodox Christian Fasting:** Many Orthodox Christians follow a fasting schedule that involves abstaining from meat and dairy on specific days, which is believed to cleanse the body and mind.

- **Ramadan in Islam:** This month-long daily fasting period promotes discipline and mindfulness around eating. The pre-dawn and post-sunset meals are generally light, reinforcing moderation.

These practices align with the findings of modern studies on intermittent fasting and autophagy—a cellular process that cleans out damaged cells.

Extended fasting periods encourage autophagy, which has been shown to reduce inflammation and improve metabolic health, potentially explaining why so many fasting traditions are linked with longevity.

Ayurveda's Take on Longevity: Eat with the Sun and Avoid Extremes

Ayurveda, India's ancient health system, offers insights into food habits and daily routines that align closely with the principles seen in long-living cultures. According to Ayurvedic texts like the Charaka Samhita, eating two meals per day—spaced around sunrise and sunset—is ideal for digestion and health. The recommendation is to eat the biggest meal at noon when the sun is above our head and eat second small, warm meal (if at all) before sunset. This pattern was believed to allow ample time for the body to digest and absorb nutrients fully before the next meal.

Some core Ayurvedic practices include:

- **Seasonal and Dosha-Based Diets:** Ayurveda suggests that food should be chosen based on individual constitution (or "dosha") and seasonal availability. This personalized approach helps balance the body's energy and reduces stress on the digestive system.

- **Mindful Eating:** Ayurveda emphasizes eating slowly and mindfully, without distractions, as this supports better digestion and absorption.
- **Daily Routine (Dinacharya):** Ayurveda prescribes a structured daily routine that includes early rising, moderate exercise, meditation, and healthy eating habits. These practices promote balance and longevity by aligning with the body's natural rhythms.

The Common Denominators: What Science Says About Long-Living Cultures

So, what's the big takeaway from these cultures that seem to have unlocked the code to a long and healthy life? Here are a few key factors:

- **Whole Foods and Low Meat Intake:** A diet based on vegetables, whole grains, and legumes, with minimal processed foods and sugar, appears to support longevity.
- **Built-In Movement:** Physical activity isn't forced; it's built into their lifestyle, whether through farming, walking, or daily chores.
- **Fasting and Digestive Rest:** Regular fasting or meal spacing allows the body to repair itself, a finding supported by modern studies on fasting's effects on metabolism and cellular health

Chapter 6: The Rhythm of Nourishment: Feeding, Fasting, and the Metabolic Journey

Let's dive into what happens inside our bodies after we eat. We'll focus on the first 72 hours of fasting (consuming only water, green tea, black coffee).

Specifically, we'll explore how the body processes the food we consume and how it shifts gears to generate energy once the food supply stops. This journey through our inner workings will reveal the remarkable systems that keep us fueled and functioning.

Introduction: Welcome to the Metabolic Marathon

From the moment we take our first bite of food, a cascade of processes begins, transforming what we eat into fuel. But once that meal is digested, the real magic starts. Over hours—and even days—our bodies go through phases of using, storing, and finally rationing energy. This chapter dives deep into that cycle, showing how our bodies handle glucose, insulin, glycogen, fat storage, and even something called "ketones" as time ticks on.

We'll follow a journey through feeding and fasting, exploring what happens every few hours, so you can see why that late-night snack might actually be delaying a fascinating—and powerful—biological process.

Welcome to Digestive Disneyland (0–4 Hours)

You've eaten! Whether it was a towering pile of pancakes drowning in syrup, a gourmet salad (that you probably had to talk yourself into ordering), or a mystery casserole, your digestive system doesn't judge—it just gets to work. For the next four hours, your body is like a high-tech factory, processing raw materials (a.k.a. food) into usable energy. This isn't just science; it's culinary alchemy, transforming that meal into three key energy sources: **glucose, amino acids, and fatty acids.**

Let's take a behind-the-scenes tour of this internal extravaganza—think of it as visiting Digestive Disneyland, where your body's processes are the real attractions.

Carbohydrates: Quick, Thrilling, and Over Before You Know It

Carbohydrates are the thrill-seekers of your meal, going full-speed from your plate to your bloodstream. The minute carbs hit your stomach, enzymes (like amylase) start working like ticket-takers at a theme park, breaking down those carbs into simple sugars, primarily **glucose**. Glucose is your body's main source of quick-burn energy, like a sugar rocket fueling your body's engines.

Once glucose enters your bloodstream, the pancreas sends out **insulin**—a hormone that's part traffic cop, part nightclub bouncer. Insulin's job? To escort glucose into your cells so they can use it as fuel. Think of insulin as the person making sure everyone gets to the right rollercoaster without causing chaos. Your brain, muscles, and organs jump on board, and suddenly you're energized and ready to tackle your next meeting, a walk, or even a nap (more on that later).

Proteins: Hard Hats Required

While carbs are zipping through your system, **proteins** are quietly breaking down into **amino acids**. These molecules are the construction workers of your body, tasked with repairing tissues, building enzymes, and creating hormones. Unlike carbs, proteins aren't in a rush to be burned for energy. Instead, they're focused on long-term projects like keeping your muscles strong, your skin smooth, and your immune system functional.

Picture amino acids as little workers in hard hats, hustling around your body to patch up cellular potholes and reinforce your biological infrastructure. They don't ask for recognition—they're the unsung heroes, keeping everything running smoothly.

Fat: A Slow, Scenic Journey

Finally, we arrive at the **fats**, the slowest of the three energy sources. While carbs sprint and proteins build, fats are your body's version of a rainy-day fund. They take their sweet time to break down into **fatty acids** and **glycerol**, which then get absorbed into your bloodstream.

Fats are a bit like the chill person at a party who knows they're not needed right away but sticks around just in case things get out of hand. Once processed, fats are stored as energy reserves, ready to step in when you've run out of glucose and need some backup power. Your body loves fats for their efficiency: they're calorie-dense, long-lasting, and essential for brain health, hormone production, and cellular membranes.

Hormonal Hijinks: Insulin's Big Moment

Here's where things get interesting. After a meal, **insulin** takes center stage, ensuring that glucose, amino acids, and fatty acids all end up where they're needed. But insulin doesn't just stop at distribution—it also handles storage.

When there's more glucose than your cells need for immediate energy, insulin cleverly directs the excess to your liver and muscles, storing it as **glycogen**. Glycogen is essentially glucose's chill cousin who hangs out in storage, ready to step in when energy levels dip later. But glycogen storage has limits—think of it like a small garage that can only fit so many cars.

Once the glycogen garage is full, insulin switches to Plan B: converting that extra glucose into fat through a process called **lipogenesis**. This fat gets stored in your adipose tissue (a.k.a. body fat) for the next time your body runs low on fuel. It's like having a spare battery pack for your phone—convenient, but not always welcome when it starts adding weight.

Why Do I Feel Like a Sloth After Eating?

Ever eaten a big meal and felt the sudden urge to nap? That's your **parasympathetic nervous system** kicking in, also known as the "rest and digest" mode. While your digestive system works overtime, your body redirects energy away from "high-priority" tasks like staying awake and toward breaking down that food.

The result? A cozy, sleepy feeling that pairs perfectly with a couch and a Netflix binge. It's your body's way of telling you, "Hey, we're busy down here. Why don't you sit this one out?"

Fun Fact: This post-meal sluggishness is sometimes called a "food coma," but don't worry—it's totally normal. Unless, of course, you've eaten your weight in carbs, in which case you're experiencing a glucose rollercoaster that might leave you feeling sluggish and bloated.

The Big Picture: Your Body's Energy Orchestra

In the first four hours after eating, your body is like a symphony, with every system playing its part. **Carbs provide the immediate energy burst, proteins focus on repairs,** and **fats quietly build reserves** for the future. Meanwhile, insulin orchestrates the entire process, ensuring everything runs smoothly.

When this stage is complete, your body has restocked its energy supplies, repaired minor cellular damage, and stashed away extras for later. It's an intricate, finely tuned process that happens every time you eat—whether it's a gourmet meal or gas station snacks.

The Slow Burn (4–12 Hours)

Your digestive system has punched the clock and gone home, but the rest of your body is still hard at work. Now comes the **post-absorptive phase**, where your internal systems shift gears. The liver takes center stage as your energy manager, ensuring your body stays fueled even without new food coming in. This phase is less like the chaos of digestion and more like your body settling into a steady rhythm, quietly balancing the books with its existing resources.

The Liver: Your Metabolic Manager Extraordinaire

Think of your liver as the accountant of your metabolism, carefully managing your body's energy budget. With no incoming calories to process, it draws from its **glycogen reserves**—a stored form of glucose—to keep things running smoothly. This glycogen stash is like a rechargeable battery, releasing glucose gradually into your bloodstream to ensure your brain, muscles, and other vital organs have the fuel they need.

The Brain's Insatiable Appetite for Glucose

Why does your brain get VIP treatment during this phase? Because it's the biggest diva in your body. Despite being just 2% of your body weight, it hogs a staggering 20% of your daily energy intake. It doesn't care about fairness— it just demands glucose, and the liver dutifully obliges. Your brain's reliance on glucose is so intense that the liver prioritizes keeping your blood sugar stable to prevent any cognitive crashes. Think of it as a constant "fuel your brain" campaign, ensuring you stay focused, alert, and not snapping at your coworkers over minor inconveniences.

The Hunger Hormone: Ghrelin's Quiet Tap on the Door

As the liver slowly depletes its glycogen reserves, your body begins to issue gentle hunger signals. Enter **ghrelin**, the hunger hormone. At this stage, ghrelin isn't throwing a tantrum or banging pots and pans; it's more like tapping politely on the door to remind you that your energy tank isn't infinite.

How to Outsmart Ghrelin

Hydrating with water, tea, or even coffee can help quiet these early hunger cues. Your stomach often confuses thirst with hunger, so sipping on a beverage might buy you a little more time before ghrelin cranks up the volume.

Pro Tip: Hunger isn't just physical; it's also psychological. If you're used to snacking every few hours, your brain may send "hunger" signals out of habit rather than necessity. Recognizing these patterns can help you decide whether it's time to eat or just a case of snack-FOMO.

Insulin Exits Stage Left, Glucagon Steps In

With no fresh food to process, **insulin**—the hormone that managed the digestion party earlier—bows out gracefully. But the show must go on, and **glucagon** takes the mic as the new hormonal star.

What Does Glucagon Do?

Glucagon's job is to signal the liver to keep releasing glucose from its glycogen reserves. This handoff from insulin to glucagon is like a seamless baton pass in a relay race, ensuring that blood sugar levels remain stable even without new food entering the system.

While insulin stores excess glucose after meals, glucagon does the opposite, encouraging the release of stored glucose to keep your body energized. It's teamwork at its finest—your hormonal system working together to ensure you don't crash and burn.

The Brain's Monopoly on Energy

Here's the thing: your muscles and other tissues are happy to start thinking about alternative energy sources, but not your brain. The brain is glucose's biggest fan and refuses to consider other fuels—at least for now. This is why the liver's glucose management is so crucial during this phase.

Without enough glucose, your brain starts sending out alarms that manifest as brain fog, irritability, or a general sense of "I need food, and I need it now." Luckily, the liver is well-equipped to handle this until glycogen reserves start running low.
Fun Fact: If you've ever felt "hangry" (hungry-angry), it's probably because your brain is freaking out over declining glucose levels. It's not subtle about its needs.

What Happens When Glycogen Runs Low?
The liver's glycogen stores aren't infinite—they typically last **12–18 hours**, depending on your activity level and metabolic rate. As glycogen reserves dwindle, your body starts prepping for Plan B: switching to fat for fuel. But don't worry—you're not there yet.

For now, the liver is still in control, doling out glucose at a steady pace and ensuring your brain stays happy. But as the hours tick by, your body will need to start making adjustments to keep the energy flowing.

Why This Phase Matters
The post-absorptive phase is your body's first step toward energy independence. By relying on stored glycogen instead of fresh calories, it gives your digestive system a break and keeps your metabolism ticking along efficiently.

This phase is also a lesson in balance. Your body seamlessly transitions from digesting food to managing its internal energy stores, showing just how adaptable and resourceful it can be. It's like a well-oiled machine, quietly doing its job without requiring constant input.

Fat Burning Show Begins(12–24 Hours)

Welcome to the **fat-burning show**, where your body starts tapping into its secret energy reserves. By now, your glycogen reserves—the quick-access fuel stored in your liver—are wrapping up their final performance. With glucose supplies running low, your body initiates a metabolic shift that makes fat the star of the show. This is the beginning of a fascinating transition, as your internal systems learn to rely on new energy sources.

The Fat-Burning Finale

Rolling Out the Fatty Red Carpet

When glycogen starts to run out, your body's Plan B kicks in: **lipolysis**, the process of breaking down fat stores into usable energy. This isn't just any energy—it's slow-burn, long-lasting, marathon-ready fuel. Think of it as switching from running on fast-burning matches (glucose) to lighting up a steady campfire (fat).

- **What Happens First**: Your adipose tissue (a fancy term for your fat cells) breaks down triglycerides into **free fatty acids** and **glycerol**. These molecules are then sent into the bloodstream, ready to fuel your muscles, heart, and other organs.

- **The Secret Stash**: It's like your body suddenly discovers a hidden energy pantry in the back of the metaphorical kitchen—filled to the brim with fat reserves it can now put to good use.

Fat Fuel 101

Not all tissues are thrilled about this switch to fatty acids. While muscles and the heart eagerly embrace their new energy source, your brain—the high-maintenance diva—has different preferences. It still wants glucose, and if it can't get enough, it demands a specialized alternative: **ketones**.

Ketones: The Brain's Backup Plan

When glucose supplies get scarce, your liver steps in to save the day with **ketogenesis**—a process that converts fatty acids into ketones, small molecules that can cross the blood-brain barrier. These ketones act as premium-grade brain fuel, keeping your gray matter sharp and functional even as your glucose levels dwindle.

Why the Brain Loves Ketones

- **Efficient Energy**: Ketones provide a steady, reliable energy supply without the spikes and crashes associated with glucose.
- **Neuroprotective Properties**: Research suggests ketones might reduce oxidative stress in the brain, offering potential benefits for cognitive function.
- **The Star Players**: The primary ketones include beta-hydroxybutyrate (BHB), acetoacetate, and a small amount of acetone (yes, the same

compound found in nail polish remover—but don't worry, it's safe in this context).

Fun Fact: The brain can eventually derive up to 75% of its energy from ketones during prolonged fasting or a ketogenic state. Talk about adaptability!

Adjusting to the New Normal: The Fat-Adaptation Phase

Switching from a glucose-dominated metabolism to a fat-based one is no small feat. Your body is essentially reprogramming itself to run on a completely different type of fuel. This transition, known as **fat adaptation**, doesn't happen overnight—it's more like teaching an old dog new tricks.

The Keto Flu: A Metabolic Adjustment Period

During this phase, you might experience mild symptoms, affectionately known as the **keto flu**. These can include:

- **Fatigue**: Your body is learning to unlock energy from fat, which takes a bit more effort than glucose metabolism.
- **Headaches**: A temporary side effect of fluctuating energy levels and electrolyte imbalances.
- **Irritability**: Your brain is adjusting to lower glucose availability, which can impact your mood in the short term.

What You Might Feel During the Transition

While your body is busy retooling its metabolic machinery, you might notice some physical and mental shifts.

- **Sluggishness**: Without its usual glycogen reserves, your body is temporarily low on quick-access energy. This can leave you feeling slower or less energetic.
- **Mild Cognitive Fog**: Your brain hasn't fully transitioned to ketones yet, so you might feel less sharp for a short period.
- **Steady Energy Incoming**: As ketones take over, you'll start to notice a more stable, enduring energy level—no more post-lunch crashes or sugar highs.

The Benefits of Fat Metabolism

Once your body fully transitions to burning fat, the rewards are worth the initial adjustment period.

1. Enhanced Fat Burning

Your body becomes a fat-burning machine, breaking down stored adipose tissue to meet its energy demands. This isn't just beneficial for weight management; it also helps maintain steady energy levels throughout the day.

2. Stable Blood Sugar Levels

With insulin levels low and ketones providing a steady fuel source, you avoid the spikes and crashes associated with a carb-heavy diet. This can lead to improved focus, mood stability, and fewer cravings.

3. Increased Endurance

Fat is an incredibly efficient energy source, providing more calories per gram than carbohydrates or protein. Once fat-adapted, your body can sustain physical activity for longer periods without needing frequent refueling.

Why This Phase Matters

The switch to fat-burning mode represents one of the most significant metabolic transitions your body can make. It's a testament to your body's adaptability and resilience, demonstrating how it can thrive even in the absence of regular meals.

By the end of this phase, you're no longer reliant on glycogen for energy. Instead, you've tapped into a virtually unlimited fuel source: your body's fat reserves. This metabolic flexibility isn't just a survival mechanism; it's a powerful tool for maintaining energy, focus, and overall health in the modern world.

Fat-Burning Orchestra (24–48 Hours)

By this point, your body is fully tuned to a new frequency, with **ketones leading the orchestra**. These little molecules are no longer just a backup fuel; they're now the headliners of your energy production system, ensuring your brain, muscles, and organs run smoothly. This phase isn't just about surviving without food—it's about thriving in a state of metabolic efficiency, mental clarity, and cellular renewal. Buckle up because things are about to get interesting.

Ketones: The Stars of the Show

Your liver is now a ketone factory, steadily producing **beta-hydroxybutyrate (BHB)**, **acetoacetate**, and a touch of **acetone** (don't worry, it's natural and nothing like nail polish remover). These ketones are not just efficient fuel; they're brain-boosting, inflammation-reducing, mood-enhancing wonder molecules.

Mental Clarity: The "Keto High"

As ketones saturate your bloodstream and power your brain, you might notice a profound shift in mental function. Tasks that once felt tedious now seem manageable. That foggy feeling? Gone. You're running on mental "high-octane" fuel.

- **Sharper Focus**: Ketones provide a steady energy source for your brain, eliminating the ups and downs caused by fluctuating blood sugar.
- **Mood Boost**: The stability ketones bring doesn't just enhance cognition—it also stabilizes your mood. You may find yourself feeling calm, focused, and even, dare we say, cheerful.

Fun Fact: The term "keto high" is more than hype. Ketones, particularly BHB, have been shown to reduce oxidative stress in the brain, supporting neurotransmitter function and making everything from creative thinking to problem-solving feel smoother.

Hunger Takes a Back Seat

With ketones flooding your system, hunger is no longer the boss of you. **Ghrelin**, the hormone responsible for those hunger pangs, starts taking a break. This appetite suppression makes fasting feel less like deprivation and more like an empowered choice.

- **No More Snack Attacks**: Instead of constantly thinking about your next meal, you might find yourself cruising through your day without the usual distractions of hunger.
- **Metabolic Efficiency**: Ketones are so effective at providing energy that your body doesn't feel the need to demand more fuel through food cravings.

Pro Tip: This is the perfect time to harness your focus and productivity. Without hunger interrupting your flow, you can tackle your to-do list—or finally dive into that novel you've been meaning to write.

Autophagy: Your Body's Spring Cleaning Service

As digestion steps aside, your body's cellular housekeeper—**autophagy**—takes the stage. Think of autophagy as Marie Kondo on a mission: damaged proteins, broken-down organelles, and cellular junk are identified, recycled, and removed.

How It Works

- **Cellular Recycling**: During autophagy, your cells enclose their damaged parts in a membrane (an autophagosome), which then fuses with a lysosome—the cell's waste-disposal unit. What emerges is a revitalized, efficient cell ready to work harder for you.
- **Energy Conservation**: With no food to digest, your body conserves energy by repurposing old

cell components instead of creating new ones from scratch.

Why Autophagy Matters

- **Inflammation Reduction**: By clearing out cellular debris, autophagy helps reduce inflammation throughout the body.
- **Anti-Aging Benefits**: Autophagy removes dysfunctional proteins that accumulate with age, potentially slowing the aging process and improving overall cellular health.
- **Disease Prevention**: Impaired autophagy has been linked to neurodegenerative diseases like Alzheimer's and Parkinson's. By enhancing this process, your body may reduce its risk of these conditions.

Fun Science Fact: In 2016, Dr. Yoshinori Ohsumi won the Nobel Prize in Physiology or Medicine for his groundbreaking work on autophagy. His research showed how this natural process is essential for health, longevity, and disease prevention.

The Physical and Mental Shift

What You're Likely to Feel

At this point, you're entering a sweet spot of fasting where physical and mental benefits become more noticeable.

- **Increased Energy**: Without blood sugar fluctuations, your energy feels consistent and reliable.

- **Mental Calm**: As ketones stabilize neurotransmitter activity, you might feel a sense of calm focus—perfect for deep work or creative pursuits.
- **Less Joint Pain**: Thanks to reduced inflammation, aches and stiffness may start to diminish.

Why You're Thriving

The body's ability to adapt to this new metabolic state is a testament to its evolutionary brilliance. During times of food scarcity, our ancestors relied on ketones to power their brains and bodies, allowing them to hunt, forage, and survive.

The Cellular Reset: Autophagy Meets Ketones

The combination of ketones fueling your brain and autophagy cleaning up cellular debris creates a state of biological harmony. This phase is often described as a **"reset button"** for your body—a chance to repair, rejuvenate, and optimize itself from the inside out.

The Role of Growth Hormone

Another key player in this process is **growth hormone**, which increases during fasting to:
- Preserve muscle mass.
- Support fat metabolism.
- Promote tissue repair and regeneration.

Pro Tip: Hydration remains crucial. As autophagy cleans up cellular waste, drinking plenty of water helps flush out toxins and supports this natural detox process.

What's Happening Behind the Scenes

- *Improved Insulin Sensitivity*
  With insulin levels at a steady low, your body becomes more responsive to this hormone. This can improve blood sugar regulation when you start eating again and may lower your risk of developing insulin resistance.
- *Mitochondrial Renewal*
  Autophagy also extends to your mitochondria—the energy powerhouses of your cells. Damaged mitochondria are replaced with more efficient ones, improving overall cellular energy production.
- *Enhanced Fat Oxidation*
  Your body's fat-burning capabilities are now in full swing, breaking down stored adipose tissue into energy. This is a direct route to reducing body fat while preserving muscle.

Hitting Your Stride

This stage isn't just about maintaining energy—it's about optimizing it. You're no longer running on fumes; you're running on a clean, efficient fuel that your body was designed to use in times of food scarcity.

What Makes This Phase Special

- **Sustained Energy**: Fat provides a long-lasting energy source that doesn't require constant refueling.

- **Mental Sharpness**: Ketones keep your brain humming along without the crashes associated with carb-heavy meals.
- **Cellular Longevity**: Autophagy ensures your cells are functioning at their best, paving the way for long-term health.

Anti-aging Zen (48–72 Hours)

Welcome to the pinnacle of your fasting journey—where your body's internal cleanup crew, led by the star performer **autophagy**, goes all out. At this stage, your body is operating like an elite housekeeping service, meticulously identifying and eliminating damaged cells, clearing out dysfunctional proteins, and even targeting some viruses. It's not just about feeling good; it's about cellular rejuvenation and longevity.

Autophagy: The Ultimate Detox and Repair

Autophagy, from the Greek for "self-eating," is your body's built-in maintenance system. During this phase, with digestion completely on pause, your cells go into full recycling mode. They're breaking down damaged parts, repurposing useful components, and discarding waste.

What's Happening?

1. **Damaged Protein Cleanup**
   Misfolded and damaged proteins, which can accumulate over time and lead to diseases like Alzheimer's, are broken down and recycled for new purposes.

2. **Clearing Out Cellular Junk**
   Old organelles and dysfunctional mitochondria
   are targeted, dismantled, and replaced with
   shiny new ones, ensuring your cells work at peak
   efficiency.
3. **Immune System Tune-Up**
   Autophagy doesn't just clean house—it boosts
   your immune system. By clearing out old
   immune cells and pathogens, your body is better
   equipped to fight off infections.

Brain Power: Enter Ketone Royalty

Your brain, the VIP of your body, is now being fueled
almost exclusively by **beta-hydroxybutyrate (BHB)**—the
king of ketones. Unlike glucose, which can cause energy
crashes, BHB provides a steady, reliable fuel source that
enhances both function and protection.

Neuron Supercharging

BHB fuels your neurons with unmatched efficiency,
helping them fire faster and more effectively. This leads
to enhanced mental clarity, focus, and even creativity.

- **Neuroprotection**: BHB shields your brain cells
  from oxidative stress, reducing the risk of damage
  from free radicals. It's like giving your neurons a
  suit of armor.
- **Brain-Derived Neurotrophic Factor (BDNF)**:
  BHB may boost the production of BDNF, a protein
  that supports neuron growth and connectivity.
  This is like Miracle-Gro for your brain, enhancing
  memory, learning, and overall cognitive health.

Cognitive Clarity and Creativity

By this point, you might notice tasks that usually feel mentally draining are now easier. The dreaded "brain fog" is gone, replaced by a sense of calm focus.

- **The "Keto High"**: Many fasters describe this mental clarity as a "keto high"—a state of heightened awareness and productivity that feels almost meditative.

Mood Boost: Calm, Cool, and Collected

Fasting isn't just transforming your body; it's stabilizing your mind. With blood sugar swings eliminated, your mood evens out, leaving you feeling grounded and less reactive to stress.

What's Responsible?

- **Ketones as Mood Stabilizers**
  Ketones, especially BHB, interact with neurotransmitters like **GABA** (calming) and **serotonin** (uplifting), creating a balanced, zen-like mental state.
- **Reduced Inflammation**
  Chronic inflammation can affect your mood and mental health. Autophagy's cleanup of inflammatory compounds helps your body and brain feel lighter and less burdened.
- **Enhanced Emotional Resilience**
  Without the rollercoaster of sugar highs and lows, your emotions stabilize. You may notice you're more patient, focused, and better equipped to handle challenges.

Hunger? What Hunger?

By this phase, hunger has pretty much left the building. The ketones coursing through your bloodstream actively suppress **ghrelin**, the hormone responsible for hunger signals.

Why Hunger Takes a Back Seat

- **Efficient Fuel**: Ketones provide such steady energy that your body doesn't feel the need to demand more food.
- **Metabolic Flexibility**: Your body is fully adapted to burning fat and ketones, so it no longer relies on constant glucose intake to function.

Pro Tip: This is a great time to embrace productivity or dive into a passion project—without hunger distracting you, you can stay in the zone for hours.

Cellular Renewal: A Full-Body Upgrade

With autophagy and ketosis working in tandem, your body is getting a serious upgrade. Here's what's happening:

- **Mitochondrial Renewal**
  Damaged mitochondria—the "power plants" of your cells—are replaced with newer, more efficient ones. This means better energy production and less oxidative stress.
- **Longevity Benefits**
  Autophagy reduces the accumulation of cellular junk that contributes to aging, promoting healthier, longer-living cells. This process has been linked to increased lifespan in studies on

animals and may offer similar benefits to humans.

- **Anti-Aging Effects**
  The combination of reduced inflammation, cellular renewal, and enhanced mitochondrial function contributes to smoother skin, improved energy, and an overall sense of vitality.

Fasting: The Superpower You Didn't Know You Had

Fasting isn't just about skipping meals—it's about unleashing your body's ability to heal, repair, and optimize itself. During this phase, your body is:

- **Burning Fat Like a Pro**: Lipolysis and ketone production are at full throttle.
- **Cleaning House**: Autophagy is repairing cells, eliminating junk, and boosting immunity.
- **Sharpening Your Mind**: BHB is powering your brain, enhancing focus, mood, and creativity.

What to Expect at This Stage

- **Physical Sensations**
  - You may feel lighter, less bloated, and more energetic.
  - Joint pain or stiffness might noticeably improve as inflammation subsides.
- **Mental Perks**
  - Your focus and problem-solving skills are at an all-time high.
  - Stress feels manageable, and you may even feel an uplifting sense of gratitude or calm.

- **Emotional Growth**
  - With hunger no longer driving your actions, you may feel a sense of control and empowerment.

Simple Summary: Body through Fed and Fasting phases

Time Period	Processes and Effects
0-4 Hours After Eating	Digestion occurs, blood sugar rises, and insulin is released to use or store glucose. Immediate energy needs are met, and excess glucose is stored as glycogen or fat.
4-12 Hours	Blood sugar and insulin levels drop as glucose intake stops. The liver begins releasing stored glycogen to maintain stable blood sugar. Gentle hunger signals may appear.
12-24 Hours	Liver glycogen is mostly used up, prompting the body to start breaking down fat for energy. Fatty acids fuel some organs, and the liver produces ketones for the brain.
24-48 Hours	Full ketosis achieved; body runs on fat and ketones instead of glucose. Brain uses ketones, leading to mental clarity and steady energy. Hunger often decreases.

48-72 Hours	Autophagy (cellular cleanup) ramps up, breaking down damaged cells for recycling. Growth hormone increases to preserve muscle. Enhanced mental clarity and reduced hunger.
By 72 Hours	Body is in a stable fat-burning state with reduced inflammation and enhanced cellular repair. Fat fuels the body, ketones support brain function, and hunger is minimal.

Supplements 101: Fasting Essentials for 72 Hours

A 72-hour fast? Your body's got it covered, but here's a quick guide to staying balanced and comfortable.

Must-Haves: Electrolytes

- **Sodium, Potassium, and Magnesium**: Essential to prevent dizziness, fatigue, and muscle cramps. Just a pinch of salt in water or an electrolyte supplement (no sugar!) will keep you steady.

Optional Helpers

- **Multivitamin**: Nice to cover any gaps.
- **Magnesium**: Great for muscle cramps.
- **B Vitamins**: If you're active, these can support energy.

Skip These

- **Antioxidants**: They interfere with autophagy, your body's natural "cell-cleaning" process, so let your body handle it on its own.

Risks to Watch For

- **Electrolyte Imbalance**: Keep hydrated and add electrolytes.
- **Dehydration**: Water is your best friend.
- In short, a bit of water, salt, and light electrolytes are your go-to's for fasting safely and smoothly.

Chapter 7: Mathematics of Fasting

Now we know that fat stored around your body will be used *only after* using up the glucose in your blood stream and glycogen in your liver.

Here is nerdy but fun science of fasting. Let's calculate weight loss from Glycogen and Fat during fasting.

Let's calculate weight loss during fasting for a 40-year-old man who is 5'10" tall, weighs 250 pounds. Fast starts after eating a regular meal.

Step 1: Calculate Basal Metabolic Rate (BMR)
The **Mifflin-St Jeor equation** is used to calculate the Basal Metabolic Rate (BMR), the number of calories burned at rest:

$$BMR = 10 \times weight\ (kg) + 6.25 \times height\ (cm) - 5 \times age\ (years) + 5$$

For our example:
- Weight: *250 lbs×0.453592 = 113.4 kg*
- Height: *(5×30.48)+(10×2.54) = 177.8 cm*
- Age: *40 years*

Substituting into the formula:
$$BMR = (10 \times 113.4) + (6.25 \times 177.8) - (5 \times 40) + 5$$
$$BMR = 1134 + 1111.25 - 200 + 5 = 2050.25\ calories/day$$

This man's BMR is **2,050 calories/day**. During fasting, body reduces energy expenditure by about 15%.

Step 2: Energy Sources During Fasting
During fasting:
- **Glycogen First:** The body burns glycogen for energy in the first 12–24 hours.
- **Fat Burning Begins:** As glycogen stores deplete, fat becomes the primary energy source.

Step 3: Energy Burn Over 24, 48, and 72 Hours
We'll calculate the weight loss assuming:
- Calories burned are adjusted for fasting: *BMR×0.85.*
- **Glycogen stores** hold **~500 grams** of energy (~2,000 calories at 4 calories/gram).
- Fat provides **~3,500 calories per pound.**

Day 1 (0–24 Hours)
- **Energy Use:** Primarily glycogen.
- **Calories Burned:**
  2050×0.85=1,742 calories
- **Glycogen Burned:** At 4 calories/gram:
  1742 calories/4 calories/gram=435.5 grams of glycogen
- **Weight Loss from Glycogen:**
  435.5 grams/453.592=0.96 lbs.

Day 2 (24–48 Hours)
- **Energy Use:** Fat becomes the primary energy source as glycogen depletes.
- **Calories Burned:** *Another 1,742 calories*

- **Fat Loss:** At 3,500 calories/lb of fat:
  1742 calories/3,500 calories/lb=0.50 lbs of fat

Day 3 (48–72 Hours)

- **Energy Use:** The body continues to burn fat for energy.
- **Calories Burned:** *Another 1,742 calories*
- **Fat Loss:** Another
  1742 calories/3,500 calories/lb=0.50 lbs of fat

Step 4: Total Weight Loss

- **Day 1:** *0.96 lbs (glycogen)*
- **Day 2:** *0.50 lbs (fat)*
- **Day 3:** *0.50 lbs (fat)*

Total Weight Loss: 0.96 + 0.50 + 0.50=1.96 lbs.

Key Insights

- **Glycogen Depletion Dominates Early Fasting:** Most weight loss during the first 24 hours comes from glycogen.
- **Fat Burning Takes Over:** After glycogen depletes, fat loss becomes steady.
- **Hydration Balances Water Weight loss:** Proper hydration ensures weight loss only from glycogen and fat.

Note: For Women, BMR equation is:
BMR=10×weight (kg)+6.25×height (cm)–5×age (years)–161

Chapter 8: A-Ha moment and Hard Truths

The A-Ha Moment: When I realized that

<u>My Body is a Fat Hoarder Prepping for the Apocalypse!</u>

Eureka!

My body sees every calorie that passes my lips as a precious resource. Anything extra? Straight to storage! A few too many cookies? Stored. That extra helping of pasta? Saved for later. Every bite that wasn't immediately necessary got tucked away in what I like to call my "Just-in-Case-of-Famine-Fund"—except, this fund doesn't have interest; it just has layers.

My body wasn't just any old saver, though; it was a *strategic* saver. It decided the best place to stash all this fat was around my organs, wrapping them up like it was trying to keep them warm for winter. Fat around my waist, fat under my skin—like bubble wrap for my insides, in case of an emergency.

Now, here's where it gets interesting. I realized that my body treats fat as its prized possession, only to be used as a *last resort*. Not only does it store every bit of excess food, but it's also *super reluctant* to ever actually *use* it. I mean, if I'm feeding it daily, my body's got no reason to dip into its precious reserves.

To make matters worse, my body has a whole list of tricks to avoid touching those fat reserves. It's got some impressive strategies: slowing down my metabolism, making me feel hungrier, or even making me feel tired to avoid using any of that stored energy. My body is basically saying, "Oh, you want me to burn fat? Nah, let's just slow things down and wait this out!"

So, there it was, my big "A-ha!" moment: to actually *use* my fat, I'd have to force my body's hand by going without food long enough to make it dip into the reserves. And if I keep eating more than my body needed, I'd be adding to the stash forever. No wonder losing fat and keeping it off is like trying to get your grandma to throw away her old Tupperware—it's just not going to happen unless you make it *absolutely necessary*.

I finally understood why my body is a bit of a fat hoarder.

Beyond this A-Ha moment, I also realized some other hard truths while doing this research and contemplating the meaning of all this.

Hard Truths:

1. **A-ha Moment: Fat is stored for a famine, and unless you go for an extended period without food, it will not be used.**
   "Turns out my body's a doomsday prepper, storing fat like canned goods for the apocalypse, and unless I fast, that 'emergency stash' isn't going anywhere!"
2. **Our body has two fuels: Glucose (readily available) and Ketones (only after extended fasting).**
   "My body's got a favorite fuel (glucose) and a VIP reserve (ketones) it only breaks out after I starve a bit
3. **Our brains work far more efficiently and with clarity on ketones than on glucose.**
   "Brain on ketones? Laser-focused genius. Brain on glucose? Let's just say it's running on battery saver mode!"
4. **Fasting is the primary lever for fat and weight loss, with exercise, reduced stress, ample sleep, and the right nutrition important but minor levers.**
   "Turns out fasting is the fat-loss MVP, while the rest are just the supporting cast—sorry, treadmill!"
5. **It is OK to stop eating when we feel full (it's better to waste food than pack it on your body).**
   "Better to trash (or refrigerate) that last bite than let it live rent-free on my hips for the next decade!"
6. **Humans follow circadian rhythm as much as plants and animals; our body's metabolism and digestive capability (Agni in Ayurveda) follows the sun, peaking at noon.**
   "Who knew? My digestion is basically solar-

powered, and it's brightest at lunchtime—no wonder dinner sits like a rock!"

7. **Don't eat when you are not hungry.**
    "Why am I eating when I'm not hungry? Because the fridge called my name? Time to hang up!"
8. **Switch celebratory meals from dinner to lunch.**
    "Swap dinner parties for lunch fiestas—your digestion (and tomorrow morning's energy) will thank you

Chapter 9: What does it all mean? Let's talk about the 'How' of weight loss and healthy living...

The goal of this book has been to equip you with the knowledge and tools you need to take control of your weight loss and overall health—without relying on gimmicks, fad diets, prescription drugs, or meal subscription plans. You don't need to follow a strict "Weight Loss Diet," jump on the Keto bandwagon, or embrace extreme intermittent fasting schedules to see results.

Instead, use a set of **Weight Loss Dials** at your disposal:

Weight Loss Dials

- Fasting Window
- Number of Meals
- Timing of Meals
- White Carbs
- Exercise
- Sleep
- Stress

Each day, you can adjust these dials to fit your unique circumstances. Over time, by consistently optimizing these dials, your body will naturally shed excess weight and become healthier.

The Power of the Dials

Fasting Window

This is the most impactful dial for weight loss. If you want to lose a significant amount of weight quickly, turn this dial up. For example:

- **Accelerated Weight Loss:** Do 24-hour fasts several times a week, with one 72-hour fast each month.
- **Gradual Weight Loss:** Fast for at least 14 hours each day (or longer when possible) and limit yourself to 2–3 meals in the remaining window.

Number and Timing of Meals

Once your fasting window is set, the number and timing of meals become key.

- For faster results, eat just **one meal a day**.
- Alternatively, eat **two meals**, such as breakfast and lunch or lunch and a light, warm dinner.

White Carbs

Avoid white bread, white rice, pasta, sugar, and potatoes for the best results. If you must have them, consume them in moderation.

Exercise

Include at least 30 minutes of walking daily and some resistance training to strengthen muscles and boost metabolism.

Sleep

Aim for a minimum of six hours of sleep to support recovery, hormone regulation, and weight loss.

Stress

Incorporate stress-management practices like meditation, journaling, or self-reflection to maintain mental clarity and hormonal balance.

Why This Approach Works

You now understand that your body is a finely tuned machine, shaped by millions of years of evolution. You've learned how excess calories are stored, why the body creates fat reserves, and when it decides to use them. With this knowledge, you can make informed, day-to-day adjustments to these dials, tailored to your unique context, instead of committing to unsustainable diets.

By tweaking these dials effectively, weight loss and improved health will follow naturally.

Practical Scenarios

- On calm, non-stressful days, turn the fasting dial way up
    - Try eating one meal a day or fasting for 48–72 hours.
    - This can result in losing 3–5 pounds per week.

- On stressful or demanding days
  - Fast for a smaller 12–14 hours.
  - Eat 2–3 balanced meals in the remaining window.

The key is to focus on **average progress** over weeks and months, rather than obsessing over daily results.

Lifetime of Results

Weight loss doesn't follow a straight, predictable path—it ebbs and flows with life. There are events, stress, parties, and travel to navigate. As you lose weight, your calorie needs decrease, and the process evolves. If you have significant weight to lose, progress tends to be faster at the beginning. Longer and more frequent fasting can accelerate weight loss, as can limiting white carbs and reducing the number of meals.

That said, gradual weight loss is perfectly fine and healthy if your body allows it. The key is understanding the levers you can control and using them effectively. This approach empowers you with the knowledge of *how*, *why*, and *when* your body stores fat. By aligning your lifestyle with your body's genetic design, you can not only lose weight but sustain it, building a foundation for a healthier life.

"Morning Metrics: Your Daily Health Snapshot"

Want to get to know your body better? No, not in a "look in the mirror" kind of way—this is about getting the hard facts straight from the source. Each morning, right after you roll out of bed (before coffee, even), take five simple measurements: Blood Pressure, Weight, Blood Sugar, Sleep Quality (how many hours you got), and Resting Heart rate. Grab an Excel sheet, set up columns for each metric and a date column, and start logging these numbers every day. And if you don't have access to a computer, just log it on paper (or your diary/journal). It's like keeping a diary for your body, but without the teenage angst. Over time, this routine not only helps you understand your baseline but also reveals patterns— what works, what doesn't, and how yesterday's choices impact today's results.

For example, wake up with elevated blood sugar? Skip the pancakes and consider a low-carb day with fewer meals to stabilize things. Feeling fatigued after a lousy night of sleep? That resting heart rate might nudge you to go easy on workouts and caffeine today. This habit helps you plan your day smarter and, over time, teaches you what your body loves (and what it silently resents). It's like being your own health detective, armed with data instead of hunches.

Simple Tracking:

Date	Weight	Sugar	Blood Pressure	Sleep	Resting Heart Rate

Weight: Get a good weighing scale. You don't need a fancy one with BMI calculations etc. BMI can be easily calculated with your height and weight.

Blood Pressure: There are many wrist BP measurement devices available for less than 40$. Any simple one will do.

Sugar: You may or may not be diabetic. I would still suggest you prick your finger every morning. It is simple once you get used to it. The devices are affordable.

Sleep: No need for a device. Just record the total sleep time.

Resting Heart Rate: If you have a smart watch that can detect heart rate, this is readily available. If you don't, just record your heart rate. It is simple to figure out without any device. Just feel the pulse at your wrist and count the number of beats in 60 seconds.

Chapter 10: The Final Weigh-In: What It All Comes Down To

So, here we are at the finish line. You've slogged through chapters packed with science, history, humor, and probably more mentions of insulin than you ever thought possible. You've learned that your body isn't a rebellious teenager ignoring your weight loss plans—it's a finely tuned survival machine doing exactly what it was designed to do. The good news? Now you know how to work with it instead of fighting it.

This chapter isn't here to give you another motivational speech (you've heard enough of those). Instead, let's tie everything together with the practical, informed approach that makes this book different. Because real, lasting change doesn't come from flipping your life upside down. It comes from understanding your body and making small, meaningful adjustments—one dial at a time.

Your Body Loves a Plan

Weight loss isn't about perfection. It's about consistency and balance. Create a flexible framework that fits your lifestyle:

- Experiment with fasting windows and feeding times to let your body tap into its natural rhythms.
- Choose nutrient-dense foods that nourish your body while keeping hunger in check.

- Embrace movement—not as punishment, but as a celebration of what your body can do.

Remember, your body is like a well-trained dog: it'll follow the routine you set, but it needs time and patience to adapt.

Master the Dials, Not the Switches

The beauty of this approach is that you're not stuck with all-or-nothing decisions. You can adjust the dials based on what's happening in your life. Stressful week? Dial back on fasting but keep your meals nutrient-dense. More time for exercise? Increase your movement dial and feel the difference. Weight loss isn't a sprint—it's a marathon where you control the pace.

Data Is Your Friend (But Don't Obsess)

The tools you've gained in this book—monitoring hunger signals, understanding hormones, and using fasting strategically—are powerful because they're grounded in evidence. But don't fall into the trap of obsessing over every calorie or step. Use data as a guide, not a drill sergeant.

Celebrate Progress, Not Perfection

Here's the truth: there's no such thing as the perfect diet, the perfect body, or the perfect lifestyle. Progress is messy, and that's okay. Celebrate the small wins— choosing water over soda, nailing a 12-hour fast, or finally understanding what leptin does (seriously, it's not that complicated anymore, right?). Every step forward is a victory.

Closing Thoughts: Rewrite Your Story

This journey isn't about perfection—it's about progress. By understanding your body and respecting its evolutionary design, you can achieve health on your terms. The weight of the matter isn't just physical; it's the knowledge that sets you free. Now, let's go rewrite your story

References

1. **Guyton, A.C., & Hall, J.E.** - *Textbook of Medical Physiology*
   Comprehensive exploration of glucose metabolism, glycogen storage, and physiological adaptations during fasting.
2. **Cahill, G.F. Jr.** (2006) - *Fuel Metabolism in Starvation*
   Annual Review of Nutrition, 26, 1-22.
   Detailed discussion of the body's transition through glycogen, fat, and ketone use during starvation.
3. **Volek, J.S., & Phinney, S.D.** - *The Art and Science of Low Carbohydrate Living*
   Examines ketone production, fat reliance during fasting, and metabolic adaptations.
4. **Berg, J.M., Tymoczko, J.L., & Stryer, L.** - *Biochemistry*
   Explains biochemical processes related to glucose, amino acids, and fatty acids during fasting.
5. **Martinez-Lopez, N., et al.** (2015) - *Autophagy and Intermittent Fasting: Effects on Aging and Disease*
   Investigates how intermittent fasting boosts autophagy and supports health.
6. **Klionsky, D.J., et al.** - *Autophagy in Health and Disease*
   Discusses the role and regulation of autophagy during nutrient deprivation.
7. **Longo, V.D., & Panda, S.** (2016) - *Fasting, Circadian Rhythms, and Time-Restricted Feeding in Healthy Lifespan*
   Cell Metabolism, 23(6), 1048-1059.
   Focuses on fasting mechanisms and their impact on health and longevity.
8. **Cavallini, G., et al.** (2008) - *Autophagy and Prolonged Fasting: Effects on Cellular Repair and Regeneration*
   a. Emphasizes autophagy's role during extended fasting periods.

9. **Frayn, K.N.** - *Metabolic Regulation: A Human Perspective*
    Explores human energy metabolism, including fat storage and utilization.
10. **Singh, R., & Cuervo, A.M.** (2011) - *The Effect of Fasting on Autophagy*
    Discusses fasting-induced autophagy and its cellular benefits.
11. **Deretic, V., et al.** - *Autophagy and Cellular Health*
    Reviews autophagy's therapeutic implications during fasting.
12. **"The Blue Zones: areas of exceptional longevity around the world"** by Michel Poulain, Anne Herm, and Gianni Pes (2013)
    This study identifies and analyzes regions with high concentrations of centenarians, exploring common lifestyle and environmental characteristics.
13. **McArdle, W. D., Katch, F. I., & Katch, V. L. (2010).** *Exercise Physiology: Nutrition, Energy, and Human Performance.* Lippincott Williams & Wilkins.
14. **Mifflin, M. D., St Jeor, S. T., Hill, L. A., Scott, B. J., Daugherty, S. A., & Koh, Y. O. (1990).** "A new predictive equation for resting energy expenditure in healthy individuals." *The American Journal of Clinical Nutrition*
15. https://www.discovermagazine.com/planet-earth/paleomythic-how-people-really-lived-during-the-stone-age